Marcia Willbrandt

aloe vera:
the miracle plant

aloe vera:
the miracle plant

by the editors of *Fit*

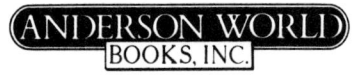

©1983 by
Anderson World Books, Inc.

*No information in this book may be reproduced in any form
without permission from the publisher.*

Anderson World Books, Inc.
1400 Stierlin Road
Mountain View, CA 94043

contents

Introduction ___ 7
History ___ 11
Getting to Its Roots ___ 16
Cosmetics ___ 20
Common Medical Uses ___ 34
Athletic Injuries ___ 39
25 Questions ___ 47
Three Case Histories ___ 55
Testimonial Letters ___ 59

aloe vera:

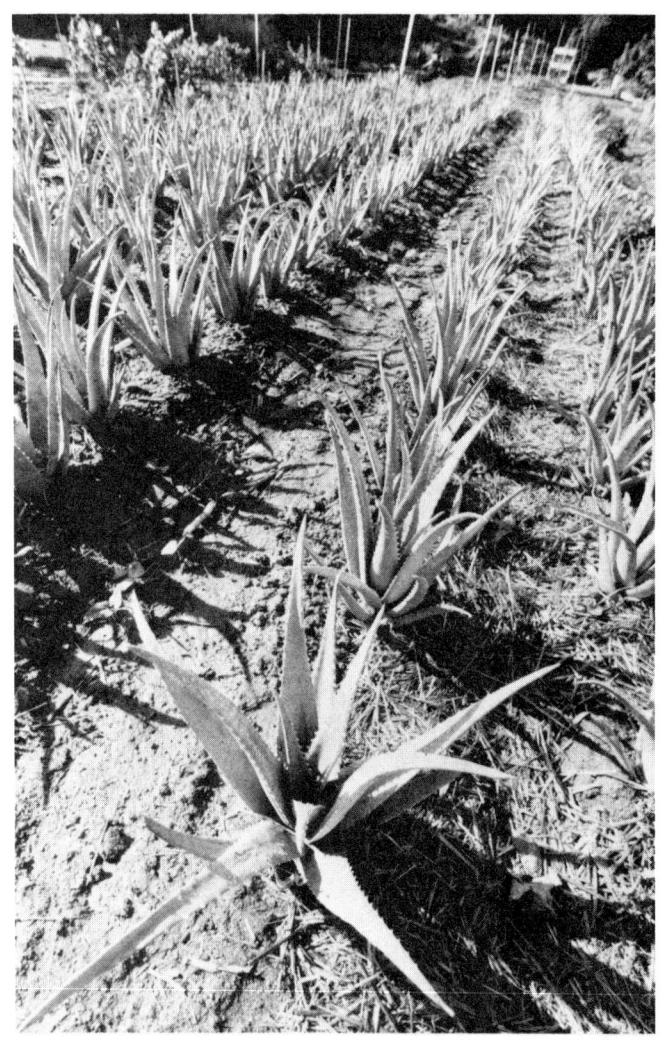

―――――――――――――――――― the miracle plant

introduction

For centuries, man has marvelled at the wonders of the Aloe Vera plant. Claims and counterclaims about its purported powers have baffled scientists, doctors, quacks and even Roman emperors. In fact, legend has it that the Roman emperors, including the notorious sex deviant, Tiberius, drank the juice of the plant to increase their sexual potency. While it may do many incredible things, it *does not* increase sexual vitality. Even though the ancient Roman chieftains were wrong — if indeed they did hold this belief — the plant served a useful purpose.

What Aloe Vera may have done for Tiberius and assorted other Romans, is provide vitamins and minerals, which compensated for an otherwise decadent lifestyle. As we now know, proper nutrition and feeling better about oneself is part and parcel of a better life, including a better sex life.

Webster's Third New World Dictionary defines aloe as,
*"a genus of succulent, chiefly southern African
plants having basal leaves with a hemplike fiber and
spicate often showy flowers."*
But it's more than that. To many people around the world, the plant offers much needed relief for the aches and pains of crippling diseases such as arthritis and other afflictions of the bones and joints. To others, Aloe Vera is one major ingredient in personal care products such as

aloe vera:

shampoos, conditioners and skin creams, among other products. The list of uses for this beautiful desert plant is endless and it will be explored in greater detail later on in this booklet. But, suffice it to say, Aloe Vera is one plant with still undiscovered — or unrecognized — potential. Both of those problems need to be challenged because it's in the best interest of the human species. There can't be a more noble cause than that.

Unfortunately, as with many new products, there is still much skepticism about the plant and its healing and cosmetic powers. This is not unusual. But it makes the need for further research and development even more critical. Some of the doubt stems from the U.S. government's licensing procedures and bureaucratic skepticism. It is all too reminiscent of Ralph Waldo Emerson's now-famous statement, "What is a weed? A plant whose virtues have not yet been discovered." This is not to imply that Aloe Vera is a weed; far from it. But there is hidden potential that needs to be tapped. The future portends many good things and chemists and other scientists are working feverishly to uncover the hidden secrets.

But even before those secrets are revealed, many people already have discovered the positive attributes of the Aloe Vera plant. Statements of personal experiences tell that side of the story. These testimonials reveal the confidence people have in Aloe Vera products and speak well for the medical and cosmetic benefits of the plant's derivatives.

The fields stretch for miles and miles in the arid Rio Grande Valley in southern Texas. One grower estimated that about four thousand acres are dedicated to the spiny, green succulent. Some people guess that many more acres than that are dedicated to the plant. As evidenced by the information in this booklet, there are numerous

the miracle plant

uses for Aloe Vera — a far cry from a report in the 1936 *Book of Knowledge:*

"Among the Mohammedans, the aloe is a symbolic plant and every Moslem, on returning from Mecca, hangs this plant over his street door as a token that he has performed the pilgrimage. In Africa, ropes, fishing lines and bow strings are made from the fiber of the leaves."

A tour of a modern Aloe Vera processing plant, many of which are conveniently located near the fields in Texas, reveals that Aloe Vera is, indeed, being used for more than a religious symbol or fishing line. The cosmetics and other products mentioned in this booklet are far more typical! Much of the Aloe Vera that goes into cosmetics comes from the leaves, which are split, and the gel inside removed.

In addition to using Aloe Vera products as a medicine or cosmetic item, there are a number of people who enjoy them as a food. One report has stated that more than one hundred thousand gallons of Aloe Vera gel are sold for external — *and internal* — use. One company we know of produces Aloe Vera jelly, which is marketed as a "pure and natural gourmet spread." It contains 33⅓ percent Aloe Vera, and flavorings ranging from papaya and honey to Jalapeno pepper.

aloe vera:

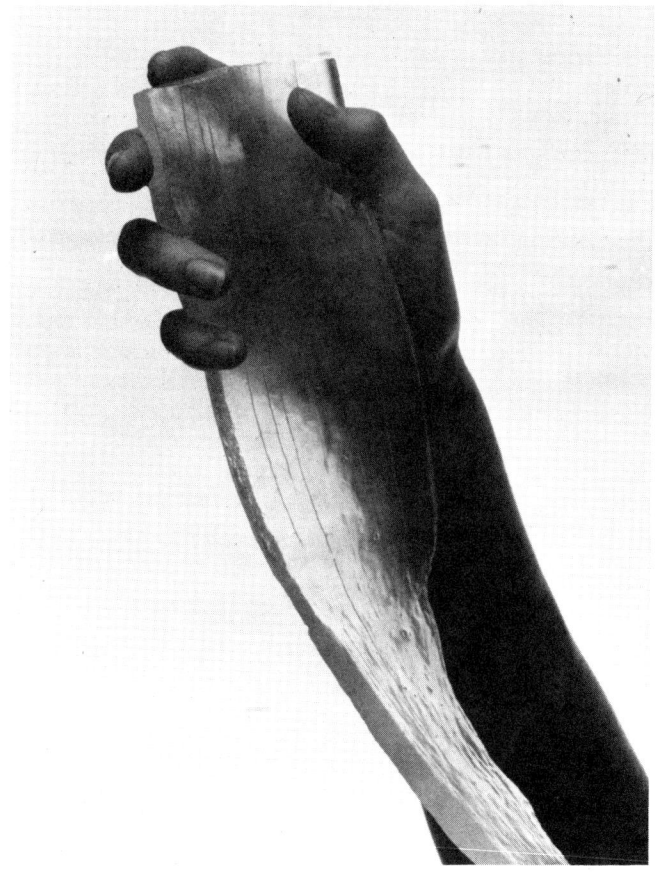

———————————————————— the miracle plant

history

> "And there came also Nicodemus which at first came to Jesus by night, and brought a mixture of myrrh and aloes about one hundred pound weight.
>
> They then took the body of Jesus and wound it in linen clothes with the spices as the manner of the Jews is to bury." John 19:30-40

Throughout history, Aloe Vera has been an extremely popular plant. Its pharmaceutical use dates far before the New Testament years of Jesus of Nazareth, probably beginning in the year 1750 B.C. A reference to it was carved into Sumerian clay tablets of that year. However, references were made to the plant — but not its uses — in ancient Egypt a couple of thousand years before the Sumerian scribe carved it into the tablet.

The Middle Eastern cradle of history, which perpetrated interest in the Aloe Vera plant, also gave it its name. The word, aloe, is a bastardization of the Arabic word for a "shining bitter substance," *alloeh*. As with many words derived from this area of the world, the ancient Hebrew pronunciation, *ahaloth,* also developed at approximately the same time.

But more than the name, the aloe plant became increasingly popular as a medicinal potient. Unlike some of the other miracle formulas developed by the ancient and

aloe vera:

medieval alchemists, though, there was something to this plant! For example, in 1550 B.C., the *Egyptian Book of Remedies* discussed various Aloe Vera plant uses. They included remedies curing infections, and the preparation of skin moisturizers and of medicines.

This is not to say that all the efforts were scientific. The Roman naturalist Pliny claimed that the ancient Egyptians used the plant products as embalming agents. There is no proof of this, however, although some believe it possible. (To this date, archaeologists have not discovered the secret of the embalming fluid that has preserved Egyptian royalty for thousands of years.)

The Arabs are credited with bringing Aloe Vera to some of the many different peoples of the Middle East. As nomads and traders, they were anxious to share some of their secrets with anyone willing to pay a price. They had mastered the art of pressing the pulp and juice from the rinds with their bare feet and, hence, are credited with its development as a drug. Among their first customers were the people of the 6th century, B.C., Persian Empire. Apparently, the extract was a popular laxative — you might say it was the early version of a well-known drug store item of modern times.

The Greeks also are credited with early research of the plant. The Greek pharmacologist, Celsus, published *De Materia Medica* in about 25 A.D. and extolled the virtues of bowel regulation with aloes. That research was continued by Dioscordes fifty years later, in 74 A.D.; he also suggested that the plant, Aloe *Vulgaris,* should be looked at as a cure for boils, bruises, chapped skin and skin abrasions, hair loss, eye sores, genital ulcers, tonsillitis and hemorrhoids.

The Romans, too, were experimenting with Aloe Vera and were amazed at some of the healing qualities of this miracle plant. Although they too recognized the plant's extracts as mainly a purgative, they also believed it would prevent hair loss when combined with wine and rubbed

the miracle plant

into the scalp. In other combinations, they believed, it had uses for these afflictions: headaches, bleeding mouth and gum, hemorrhoids and dysentary. (The latter ailment was "cured" — or so they believed — when it was applied as an enema.)

But the history of Aloe Vera is more than a lesson from the ancient past in remote areas of the Middle East or early Rome. Aloe Vera's benefits were quickly discovered by the Mayan Indians in Mexico's Yucatan Peninsula, the Seminoles of Florida and the indigenous populations of the islands of Curacao and Cuba. Where the plant and its benefits did not flourish were the countries of Northern Europe, such as Sweden and Finland; weather conditions there do not allow for the plant's development.

As a succulent, Aloe Vera can be grown almost anywhere. It thrives in the hot, desert climates of the Middle East and the Americas. It does not do well in areas characterized by long, cold winters.

But back to the warm climate of the Caribbean. The natives there experimented with many Aloe Vera uses, including as an internal potient for illness. This differed from other New World uses, which involved its application as an external (skin) medicine for ailments like blisters and insect bites. It has been reported that the priests and doctors who attended to the natives are the ones who demonstrated many of the Aloe Vera uses.

In fact, the clergy — especially the Society of Jesuits — is responsible for much of Aloe Vera's popularity. As any student of the Middle Ages and Renaissance knows, they were the best-educated people of their era. They relied on much of the information from the early researchers of Greece and Rome. Given that the preponderance of the Jesuits were from Spain and Portugal — whose climate lent itself to the cultivation of Aloe Vera — it was only logical for these men to experiment and learn from the lessons of the past. Logically, these priests who traveled to all parts of the world — and especially the new-found land in

aloe vera:

North America — would bring the best from their homeland. Because of the Jesuit knowledge of pharmacology, it was only a matter of time until the benefits of the Aloe Vera plant would be spread throughout the New World. Luckily for the natives of the Caribbean and ultimately the North and South American continents, a new form of relief was now available to help cure some of the indigenous ailments.

So, in time, Aloe Vera became an international hit. From its early roots in the days of the Old and New Testaments, to the time of Cleopatra, when she reportedly used the Aloe Vera gel (the substance inside the leaves) as a cosmetic, Aloe Vera has been acclaimed as a plant of infinite importance. Its worth is illustrated best by pointing out that in Biblical times, the nomadic people uprooted plants from the desert before moving on to another area, in the event that they found that Aloe Vera was not available in the next location.

Interestingly enough, it was not long until the ancients learned that Aloe Vera could be used both as a medicine and a cosmetic. The blistering Middle East sun and the dry desert winds had (and still have) chapping effect. It did not take a lot of experimentation to learn that aloe gel applied to the skin helped ease the burning sensation and promoted quick healing.

On the other side of the world, the Chinese advanced the idea of the sacred Aloe plant. The early Oriental physicians insisted on using Aloe Vera to heal such complaints as stomach and colon ailments. The natives of the Congo in Africa learned to use Aloe Vera from a purely practical — rather than medical or cosmetic standpoint. They would drink the Aloe Vera liquid to purge their internal systems and eliminate strong body odors. They believed this to be important in the stalking and hunting of wild animals. The Philippine people, as well, would drink the liquid — usually with their milk. This, they believed, would help alleviate dysentary and kidney problems.

the miracle plant

Although, as previously mentioned, the Jesuits are widely credited for spreading Aloe Vera throughout the New World, the first transport of it to these unexplored territories is believed to have been on Columbus' ship. Referring to its seemingly magical qualities, the crew members called Aloe Vera the "potted physician."

As its popularity spread among the North American natives, it did not take long until Aloe Vera became an important part of early American medicine. At the same time, others in the Americas — mainly in Mexico — were discovering Aloe Vera as a scalp, shampoo and hair conditioning agent. But they, too, learned that Aloe Vera had medical qualities, as well. As the Spanish settlers scattered throughout Mexico, they needed to find relief for a skin condition, *erysipelas* — a highly inflammatory bacterial infection — common in persons of Spanish origin. They learned quickly that Aloe Vera helped to relieve problems associated with this disease.

Modern man, on a wide scale, is just now reawakening to the Aloe Vera miracle. Various companies are emerging around the United States and other parts of the world to develop Aloe Vera products for both cosmetics and medicine (as well as for some other purposes). Many companies, which infuse their goods with only a small amount of Aloe Vera, rely on other chemical ingredients to work with the natural qualities of the plant. While this is not exclusive to the Aloe Vera industry — other industries are in the throes of a natural vs. synthetic controversy — it is important for the consumer to understand the differences between one Aloe Vera product and another.

aloe vera:

getting to its roots

Just what is Aloe Vera? Aloe Vera is one of hundreds of species of *Aloe*, a perennial succulent of the lily family. Although its lance-like, spiny leaves give it the appearance of a cactus, Aloe is not of that family, nor is it related to the American Aloe, or century plant. Several species of Aloe grow wild in many parts of the world. There are also several species throughout the United States, particularly in the Southwest. Aloe Vera is a popular house plant whose leaves are still occasionally used by housewives to soothe minor cuts and burns. Interestingly, a 1964 crop research report by the U.S. Department of Agriculture indicated that Aloe Vera would never be commercially profitable. Now, however, the plant is being cultivated in the Southwest to supply the growing market for Aloe Vera products.

The genus *Aloe* belongs to the lily family *(Lilaceae)*, which includes a large number of ornamental plants such as lilies, tulips and hyacinths as well as — if you can believe it — onions and asparagus. Of the hundreds of species of Aloe, only a handful have any commercial uses.

The aloe gel most often used in cosmetics is taken from the species known botanically as *A. barbandensis Miller.* The gel is a water-thin, almost colorless liquid extracted from the peeled, spineless leaves of the plant.

As a drug, aloe comes from the dried latex from the leaves of either the *A. barbandensis Miller* or of *A. ferox Miller,* or hybrids of it with two other species (*A. africana Miller* or *A. spicata Baker*).

the miracle plant

Whatever the succulent is called, it is a variation of the same plant. In Latin, the words *aloe vera,* mean "the true aloe"; there can be no greater truth than that when referring to the many varieties grown. The chemical makeup of the plant is basically the same and it is this chemistry that holds the key to the plant's many powers. While, as a succulent, the plant is composed mainly of water, the impressive list of other ingredients is best illustrated by the following chart:

ELEMENTS IN ALOE VERA GEL*

Element	Description	Benefit
Lignins	Pulp-like substance that works with cellulose to comprise leaf gel.	Thought to be able to penetrate human skin.
Saponins	Glycosides (condensation of sugar).	Cleansing and antiseptic capability. Ability to suds (important in cosmetic products).
Anthraquinones including aloin, barbaloin, isobarbaloin, anthranol, anthracene, aloetic acid, ester of cinnamic acid, aloe emodin, chrysophani acid, ethereal oil, resis tannol	The basis of a natural cathartic principle in plants.	Believed to be pain-killers; antibacterial agents.

aloe vera:

Inorganic Ingredients		
Minerals including calcium, potassium, sodium, choline, manganese, magnesium, zinc, copper, chromium	The trace elements of the human system available from the gel.	Highly interactive with vitamins to aid human functions.
Vitamins including B_1, B_2, Niacinamide, B_6, Choline, Folic Acid, C		Essential to nutrition when ingested in their proper amounts.
Mono- and polysaccharides including cellulose, glucose, mannose, aldonentose, L-rhamnose. Enzymes including oxidase, amylase, catalase, lipase, aniinase. Lysine, threonine, valine, methionine, leucine, isoleucine, phenylalanine		All work to supplement the body's own resources.

*Keep in mind that others may still be discovered.

So, that's the key. The mixture of active ingredients in aloe is obtained from the leaf's gel. They are widely believed to be responsible for Aloe Vera's healing powers. Elaborating on the information contained in the chart, the gel offers the key trace minerals so essential to life itself. For example, calcium is the key to human bone formation and the regeneration of damaged bone tissue. Sodium and potassium, the salts regulating human metabolism, are essential to the regulation of nerve impulses. A shortage of potassium, another active aloe ingredient, can

the miracle plant

cause dizziness and even fainting. Zinc levels have been linked to sexual potency (maybe the ancient Romans knew more than we thought they did about the powers of Aloe Vera), and urinary tract health and disease. An absence of manganese can cause nerve disorders, infertility and retarded growth. Lack of magnesium, found in liver tissue, can cause irritability, convulsions and can — in extreme cases — be fatal.

There's no doubt about it: The plant — and even its detractors would admit this — is rich. It's almost as though it was put on this planet to serve man's interests. It's easy to understand why the ancient people believed it to be more than just another plant and why, in some cases, it was actually worshiped by them. Few plants offer as many nutritive, medicinal and pharmaceutical, cosmetic, and tasteful (many people simply enjoy Aloe Vera's by-products as a food) benefits. Now we can reap the benefits of Aloe Vera items on every level, from medicine to cosmetic to food. Where we have it over our predecessors is the ability to manufacture an even greater number of items for a much larger populace.

aloe vera:

cosmetics

Ever since Cleopatra was made aware of the potential of Aloe Vera as a skin moisturizer, people have taken advantage of the wonderful cosmetic benefits of the plant's by-products. At the same time, consumers should know that if they want to get any benefit from Aloe Vera at all, they should look for cosmetic items with at least 70 percent Aloe Vera. When purchasing the products, make sure the face cream, hand lotion, bath gel or shampoo — among other items — contains that minimum amount of aloe. Of course, any amount will be beneficial, but the right amounts — free of chemicals and other additives — provide the cosmetic appeal. That's why you must pay close attention to the other ingredients that accompany the aloe. As a vegetable, the Aloe Vera plant can easily be polluted with other chemicals and artificial preservatives, which presents a potential danger to your skin.

Most companies, though, recognize this, and the number of different cosmetics available on the market is staggering. It's popular because of the Aloe Vera gel's unique property to penetrate deep into the skin layers — all the way to the water-retaining levels (depending on the item). This is in sharp contrast to many other cosemtic items — those without Aloe Vera — because these tend to sit on the skin without penetrating. The effectiveness, therefore, of these creams, cleansers, oils, body lotions and rubs is minimized.

the miracle plant

One beautician offered this advice to women who want to take advantage of Aloe Vera's cosmetic properties. It's a step-by-step program designed to enhance the skin:

1. Wash hands. Use a soap containing aloe, especially those with a jellied cleanser. The jellied cleanser penetrates deep into the skin and into the pores. Wash it off with a warm cloth.

2. Use an Aloe cleansing bar. There is a particular advantage for those with acne because aloe does get beneath the pores. Wash the face, neck, chest and shoulders — all the areas in which there is a potential for acne.

3. After the aloe cleansing, use an aloe skin stabilizer. This helps to stabilize the pH (acid level) of the skin, and those products with high amounts of aloe tend to work better.

4. The last step is to use an aloe moisturizing cream or lotion. Be sure to pick the one designed for your type of skin — they are available for people with dry and normal skin types.

Most, if not all, beauticians and cosmeticians would be the first to endorse daily bathing as another good way to take care of your skin. But, if improper cosmetics are used, the consequences can include dry skin and other dermatological conditions. Aloe Vera products can easily come into play here.

Baths have been regarded as one of life's luxuries, ever since they were made popular by the ancient Romans and Greeks. The Japanese have been soaking in tubs for centuries and, on the other side of the world, the Scandinavians have promoted the use of saunas. Of course, hot tubs in the 1970s were — and to some degree still are — part and parcel of California culture.

But what makes the bath so inviting to women, is that it can be an effective beauty treatment for the entire body. Depending on what you put in the water — and the list of moisturizing bath oils, gels and crystals available on the

aloe vera:

market is endless — you can either improve or not help — and maybe harm — your skin. Many products just sit on top of your skin without penetrating.

Aloe Vera products, with their ability to penetrate deeply and effectively, offer a very positive opportunity to give your skin an inviting workout. While sitting in your next bath, consider this: Aloe Vera does penetrate to the water-retaining level of the skin and when it does, the enzymes discussed earlier break down the dead cells that accumulate on the surface of the skin. That's why teen-agers and others with acne all over their bodies should take advantage of a soak in a bath of aloe oil. Reportedly, Aloe Vera has almost the same pH factor as the skin. That's why most people with terrible allergies can use the gels without adverse reactions. And this includes even the purest gels. There are numerous Aloe Vera oils available on the market and, usually, only one capful is enough to make your bath even more beneficial than it already is.

If you're shampooing, be sure to use shampoos containing Aloe Vera. After the bath, rub yourself gently with a towel and apply Aloe Vera after-bath gel.

Aloe Vera works on the hair in much the same way it does on the skin. Given that hair is an extension of the scalp, it's only logical that the effect would be similar. All human hair, like the skin itself, goes through a cycle of death and replacement. When the hair dies, the cells multiply in the papilla (a small elevation at the end of the root that is responsible for hair growth) and new hair replaces the dead hair. But, despite the fact that most people have a strong, healthy blood supply to the hair, it is affected by external conditions. Wind, sun, cold and chlorine in water, among other villains, tends to strip away the nutrition. Then come shampoos and other soaps. They really do not do the job unless they are specifically designed for the type of hair being shampooed. That's why it is so important to make the proper considerations when purchasing

the miracle plant

shampoo and cream rinses. This is especially true, given the man-made factors that help damage the hair, such as blow-drying, curling irons and other mechanical devices.

All this is why Aloe Vera in shampoo and conditioners is so important. Since it penetrates the hair follicles, and the scalp itself, it helps to open pores and cleanse the scalp, washing away the impurities. In much the way it works on skin, the amino acids present in the aloe gel penetrate the follicles and papilla and help to restore the healthy tissues.

As a conditioning agent, aloe is also very good because it penetrates the hair shaft. Aloe Vera contains a chemical composition very similar to the keratin — the substance composed of amino acids, oxygen, carbon and small amounts of hydrogen, nitrogen and sulfur, which constitutes most of a hair follicle. This is why conditioners containing Aloe Vera work so well. The hair is revitalized with its own basic nutrients. This makes the hair more elastic and thus keeps it from breaking.

How women and men use cosmetics differs from person to person. How companies manufacture cosmetics differs in much the same way. Many firms market creams and other products containing Aloe Vera. Others market the pure — or mostly pure — gel taken directly from the leaves as part of the refining process. What is important, is that a person interested in items containing Aloe Vera products understand precisely the nature of that product. One lab we know of fillets the Aloe Vera leaves and cuts off the tips and ends and sides. Then the gel — containing those all-important chemicals — is liquified and bottled. That's all the buyer gets. There are no other fancy additives. This is not to say that the additives are detrimental. On the contrary, many times the chemists who develop these products understand how important synthetic additives can be. But, as our predecessors knew, the gel itself, with nothing else in it, offers important cosmetic (and other) benefits. The purchaser of a gel product

aloe vera:

knows exactly what is being bought — there is nothing but the living vitamins and minerals.

In many cases, it is wise to seek consultation from a dermatologist, who can analyze and advise you about cosmetics. Since everyone has different types of skin, it is important — in fact, mandatory — that the appropriate cosmetic be used. Men, women, teen-agers and even babies have different needs. Since not one company can produce one product for this diverse audience, selective and educated purchasing is crucial. Older men and women, too, must recognize that skin changes with age. Therefore, what may have been appropriate in one year may not be right the next. A person in her twenties should consider one type of make-up and that should be altered in her thirties, forties and so on. Be aware of your skin and watch for tell-tale signs of problems. Dermatological nuisances such as peeling skin, blotches and extremely oily skin are only a few of the many signs that a change is necessary. Don't wait to see a doctor if you are worried. Problems can also indicate something more serious than the wrong cosmetic.

An understanding of what cosmetic to use can only happen if you fully appreciate exactly what a cosmetic is. Cosmetics encompass everything from toothpaste to bubble bath. The industry is huge. One source claims that it is the second biggest in the world, behind only the food industry. Until very recently, many companies were not paying attention to the chemical needs of the skin. Aloe Vera-producing cosmetic firms were among the leaders in this regard; that's because Aloe Vera's natural benefits immediately skyrocketed it to the forefront of the cosmetic industry. Now, everywhere you turn at the cosmetic counter, you can find products containing Aloe Vera. That's because Aloe Vera provides natural pH balancing. The gel's natural ingredients appear to offer a perfect way to cleanse and remove the bacteria and fungus that causes

the miracle plant

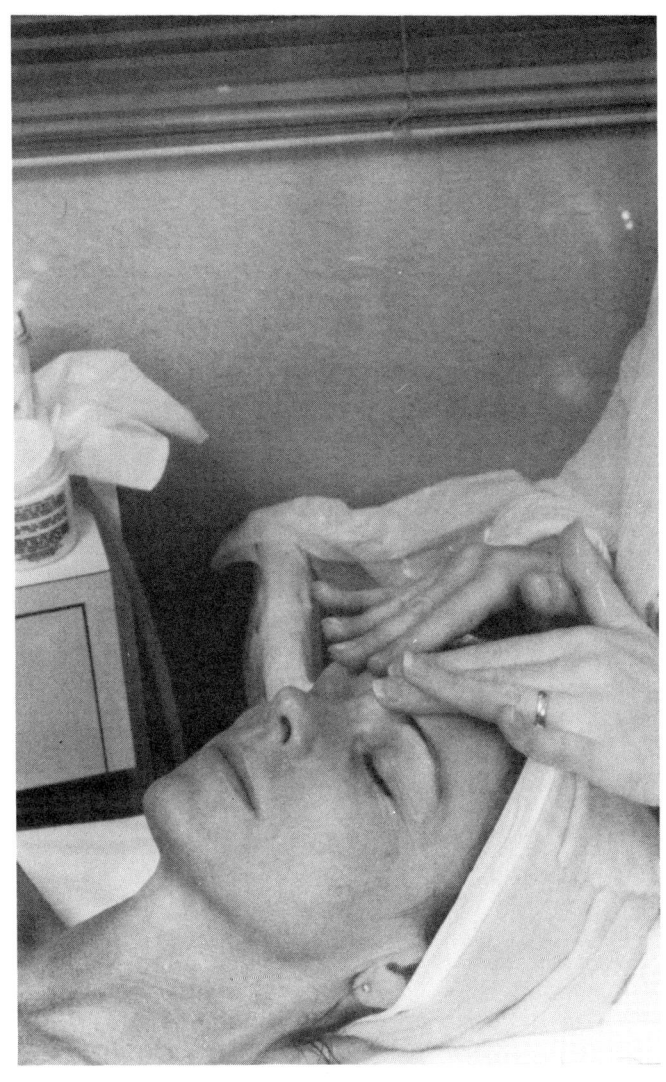

aloe veRa:

so much dermatological disruption. The deep penetrating ability of the lignins and polysaccharides is the perfect transport vehicle for the many nutrients that can feed the living cells in the dermis and hypodermis. In the same manner, the natural nutrients feed the skin. The vitamins, minerals, sugars and other essential elements are there when needed. The amino acid chemistry of the plant helps to develop new cells at an unusually rapid rate and, on the other side of the coin, the enzymes help to push off the dead cells from the epidermis. That's extremely important because it is only in this way that a natural base for new tissue can be formed. In the same way that Aloe Vera helps to provide life to dry hair, the natural ingredients of the gel help to provide moisture to the skin.

Lack of skin moisture after a day at the beach is probably one of the most painful and irritating skin conditions known. Sunburn has plagued, and continues to plague, outdoor enthusiasts. As noted in the introduction of this booklet, the ancient Egyptians quickly discovered that application of the gel could do two things: prevent sunburn and, if necessary, relieve the pains of a burn. So it is in modern times. Although most sunburns are not dangerous, they can be very painful. Immediate application of the Aloe Vera juice, gel, or ointment, provides the best results and reduces complications. If the skin is kept moist with the juice, the burn will hurt less and heal faster. As a lotion, aloe is one of the best ways to prevent sunburn.

Acne and Aloe Vera

As mentioned, it is highly beneficial to plot out a specific skin care program. In our discussion of cosmetics and make-up, a step-by-step program was recommended. But persons with definite dermatological problems should, in consultation with a physician, plan a routine and adhere to it. One of the toughest skin conditions faced by teens and many adults is acne. It shows up in four different

the miracle plant

ways. The first, as a blackhead, in the least critical form, is caused by oils and other residues in the pores. The second, as a whitehead, is an irritation and pore clogging covered by skin. As a full-fledged pimple, the pores have become blocked and are irritated, inflamed or infected. The toughest form — referred to as *acne vulgaris* — can leave disfiguring scars and permanent skin damage. This is usually caused by a variety of different types of cysts and nodules.

Here is a recommended program to fight against any or all of these conditions: 1) Wash the skin regularly with an Aloe Vera cleanser in order to remove as much bacteria and oil as possible. 2) Be sure to keep all hair brushes and combs absolutely clean at all times. 3) Get enough sleep and rest. 4) Maintain a good diet, avoiding rich and so-called "junk foods." 5) Avoid spreading infection by not touching the affected area.

Bill Coats, author of the comprehensive book about Aloe Vera (*The Silent Healer: a Modern Study of Aloe Vera*), reports many success stories related to Aloe Vera products and acne. One letter, as an example, speaks for itself:

"I have had oily skin with pimples and bumps since I was fourteen years old, and had visited many doctors over the years. My hormone problem, nerves, etc., contributed to the problem but nobody ever found anything that really cleared my face except momentarily. I literally was a middle-age teen-ager skin-wise. My sister insisted this [an Aloe Vera product] would help if I would stay with it. I did, even though it got much worse about a month after I started it... and she made me keep on, to fight all infection and heal it. It took five long months, but it worked... though I do have to work at it constantly to keep clear. I discovered the oil continues to collect... and the only solution is that I must include the Aloe Vera product on a constant basis. I am resigned to the fact that my body

aloe vera:

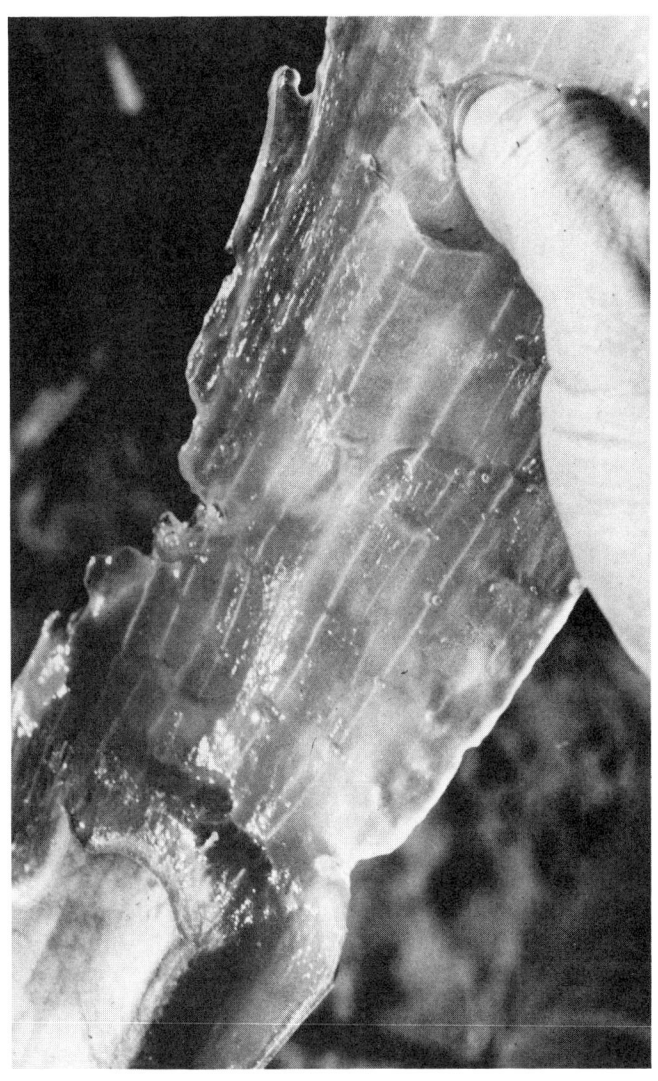

conditions will not change, giving me that skin miracle..." This writer went on to say that at least Aloe Vera products offered a "continual program not available elsewhere."

Aloe Vera Gel Nutrients That Have a Specific Cosmetic Benefit

Zinc: One of the most important minerals for healthy skin and nails.

Potassium: This is essential for maintenance of firm face and body muscles.

Iron: Carries oxygen throughout the body and especially to the cells that replenish the skin.

Vitamin A: Vital for tissue oxygenations. Without this, a person would be replete with blemishes, dry and unhealthy hair and weak toe- and fingernails.

Folic Acid: Mandatory for healthy skin and hair.

Choline: Also mandatory for healthy skin and hair.

What About Drinking Aloe Vera For Healthy Skin?

It follows that if Aloe Vera gel applied to the skin in the form of soap or conditioners is so beneficial, than the juice of the plant should provide identical benefits, which it does.

Persons on a diet can permanently damage their skin and cause harm to their nails by limiting the amount of calories that come into the body. Eventually, the body will become starved for what it previously had become used to.

Many diet doctors and other experts who advise men and women how to shed those excess pounds, will recommend the ancient Aloe Vera plant — usually in juice form — as an excellent diet supplement. Not only will those essential vitamins and minerals, which are lost in many diet programs, be maintained, but the skin and nails will be protected.

aloe vera:

Reducing fat too quickly can make skin look withered and old. That's why afflictions like rough and dry spots are so common among those who diet. In severe circumstances, such problems as non-living skin are not uncommon. It's usually noticed among the aged, but with more and more regularity, this problem is cropping up among the young, especially those who diet.

In the book *Super Skin* by Dr. Jonathan Zizmor, it was reported that an "experimental diet of one thousand five hundred seventy calories daily for twenty-three weeks resulted in poor skin with aging characteristics, plus hair that became dull and dry had a tendency to stop growing and fall out." He added that, "In young people, the damage is reversible with weight gain" but as one becomes older, it is more and more difficult.

The danger is that there is the risk of a vitamin deficiency, unless there is some sort of vitamin, mineral, amino acid or enzyme supplementary source. Without it, the damage to the skin, as mentioned, can be permanent since the skin must be nourished from the inside.

Aloe Vera juice, available commercially, is a perfect supplement for dieters. Consider drinking a minimum of about eight ounces daily for essential additions to the diet. Aside from being a refreshing low-calorie drink, the juice helps to keep the body, hair and face well conditioned. What a way to disguise the strains of a diet!

It's not only juice that offers these benefits. There are Aloe Vera vitamins on the market, which help to nourish the hair, nails and skin during a diet. One such vitamin releases vitamins and minerals plus amino acids throughout the day and night instead of all at once. However, if it's ingested — in juice or tablet form — the dieter now has another chemical-free way to better skin and good looks.

Another form of body fat, which plagues women especially, is commonly called cellulite. That rippled skin that hangs to the upper thighs, abdomen and buttocks, often refuses to go away, despite constant dieting. It's difficult to get rid of because cellulite is a gel made up of ordinary water that becomes trapped in pockets right beneath the surface of the skin. The only way to rid the body of cellulite is to plan a diet that purifies the body of excess water and wastes without forcing it to burn fat in the area in which that does not need to happen.

Among many women, cellulite is a recurring nightmare. It bulges out at the most inopportune times, in the most inopportune moments. It mostly strikes women who do not get enough exercise. But a regular exercise program is a sure way to avoid the nuisance. Women who are prone to tension, fatigue, poor breathing, lack of energy-expending exercise, polluted air and not enough fluid are the prime cellulite candidates.

It may, however, be effectively fought with a daily drink of Aloe Vera juice. Since the liquid is a natural laxative — as its ancient users knew — it rids the body of unwanted waste products. By cleansing the kidneys, sluggish digestion becomes an affliction of the past. This allows for relief of constipation and excellent circulation. Under normal circumstances, foods that have been eaten to excess do not get flushed out in total and, as a result, the extra calories work to form pockets of flesh — cellulite.

How Does The Public Know What's What In Cosmetic Products?

As mentioned a number of times in this booklet, it is extremely important to understand the percentage of active ingredients in Aloe Vera products. For reasons explained above, this is particularly important for cosmetic and medical products. But the question has been confusing to both the public and the industry itself.

It was in the summer of 1982 that the industry adapted a standard. The National Aloe Science Council (NASC) announced the development of an analytical procedure designed to determine the percentage of active ingredients contained in Aloe Vera products. The NASC issued a statement that read:

"Drs. Ivan E. Dannoff and Bill McAnalley, faculty members at Southwestern Medical School in Dallas, created the new procedure in cooperation with the NASC scientific committee. The researchers' first task was to identify a substance indigenous to aloe, yet not present in any appreciable amounts in most other plants and natural substances. In addition, the substance would be one not available commercially in a natural or synthesized form. Now that Dannoff and McAnalley have identified a substance which meets all the criteria, it is possible to compare quantities found naturally in a group of aloe leaves to the amounts present in manufactured products containing processed aloe gel extracted from those leaves.

"We believe we have found an effective analytical tool for providing quality control in the aloe industry," said the president of the NASC scientific committee.

"According to Smothers, aloe is a complex plant which undergoes certain internal fluctuations as a result of the climatic changes and natural growth cycles. The amount of active ingredients within the plant may vary by 30 to 60 percent during the year. Because of the fluctuations, Smothers and his team of researchers will attempt to isolate several other substances within the plant to serve as additional checkpoints during analysis.

"Once the analytical procedure is completely refined," Smothers said, "the NASC will attempt to write standards for aloe products using a gradient method or some other standard criterion. Our most pressing objective through this research is to promote accurate labeling for all aloe products . . ."

There is one important point to remember vis a vis this controversy. Consumers must know that products with Aloe Vera gel or products containing Aloe Vera will not be benefical until they have been stabilized — that is, they must be preserved. Without this stabilization, the properties that make Aloe Vera useful decompose and the product becomes valueless.

The other point to keep straight is differentiating between the gel and the juice, both described in this section. The gel is derived from the thin-walled cells of the leaves. It's used mainly in cosmetic preparations, but it also appears to have a strong pharmaceutical potential (more about this later). The gel itself contains a liquid that is extracted from the fibers. This liquid, when stabilized, is the aloe product sold commercially for cosmetic uses.

The juice, on the other hand, is obtained from the cells directly beneath the plant's leathery skin and it, too, has numerous cosmetic and health-related uses.

If you have any questions about the stabilization process or the effect of the Aloe Vera on your skin, be sure to consult an expert, who will explain that the stabilization process keeps the gel from becoming contaminated. The expert should also explain why it is important to look for Aloe Vera products that have not been stabilized through a heat process, which destroys the active ingredients of the plant — those important elements that offer so much.

Remember, too, that miracles do not happen overnight. Don't expect to rid yourself of acne or some other dermatological condition after just a few treatments with an Aloe Vera product. It takes time — maybe months — maybe years. And it's not a substitute for good diet, rest and exercise. A good skin and hair care plan works in coordination with a healthy lifestyle to provide the reward of healthy and good-looking skin. Aloe Vera cosmetics are truly a way to bring about a healthy and radiant appearance. But, as with anything, it all takes time, a well planned routine and persistence. We must learn from Cleopatra, who believed Aloe Vera to be only part of a total program for beauty.

aloe vera:

common medical uses

"Herbert Meents, a distributor of Aloe Vera products in Kankakee, Illinois, says he drinks a liquid containing aloe to keep his ulcers under control. Patricia Downs, a clerk in a Chicago health foods store, relies on a slushy drink that's mostly aloe to ease her spastic colon. Harry J. Melnick, a dentist in Chicago, says he switched to a new toothpaste containing aloe after it helped a patient with cigar-stained teeth and ailing gums. Other aloe fans credit the plant with curing acne, arthritis and canker sores."

Where did this quote come from? It wasn't the *National Enquirer* or a similar publication. It was, in fact, the prestigious *Wall Street Journal* in its October 6, 1982, edition. The significance of the article that appeared in the *Wall Street Journal* is obvious — Aloe Vera has finally come of age. It's being noticed. And for good reason.

We've spoken in passing about a number of the medical problems that can be attacked with Aloe Vera. We'll detail them here and try to explain why Aloe Vera is a plant that should be looked at carefully by people with certain ills.

Acne: This is one of the medical problems that can also be a cosmetic problem. That's why it was covered earlier in this booklet.

Burns: The scientific tests discussed earlier dealt, in great respect, with Aloe Vera as a vehicle to speed the healing

the miracle plant

process. Recall that the first modern use of Aloe Vera was in the laboratory for patients with X-ray burns. Since then, as mentioned, it has been used for burns derived from chemicals, to those as a result of small kitchen fires. Obviously, should you suffer a severe burn, see your physician. But until that time, it is worthwhile to consider Aloe Vera as a good form of relief. Ask your physician whether or not you should continue the Aloe Vera treatment. More often than not, he or she may advise you to go ahead with it.

Psoriasis: It appears that the antibacterial and fungicidal qualities of the stabilized Aloe Vera gel have a substantial effect on psoriasis. We know of one patient, a forty-five-year-old woman, who tried the conventional methods of treatment — cortisone cream and ultraviolet light. At least two months of treatment showed little progress. After application of an Aloe Vera cream, she noticed some clearing. Within two weeks, relief was in sight. In fact, much of the irritation and redness disappeared.

Ulcers: There are numerous cases of people who drink Aloe Vera juice or ingest the gel to cure problems with stomach ulcers. In one particular case, a farmhand in southern Texas suffered severe stomach pains, accompanied by nausea and vomiting. He consulted with his physician, who informed him that he had a bad stomach ulcer. The doctor advised treatment in a hospital, warning that if he (the patient) didn't receive immediate attention, the results could be fatal. To make a long story short, the farmhand ignored his doctors orders and began a regular program of cure involving the gel of the Aloe Vera plant. (Of course, being that he was located in southern Texas, this was relatively easy. This is the prime growing ground of the miracle plant). Now, twenty years later, he is still drinking the gel three times a day. He has not been bothered by his ulcer in years.

Dental Care: Dentists around the country are endorsing

aloe vera:

various Aloe Vera products in the treatment of mouth disorders, including canker sores, pain related to dentures and other oral afflictions.

Foot Problems: Again, the fungicidal and anti-bacterial qualities of Aloe Vera come into play. Many of the potential foot problems you can suffer respond well to Aloe Vera treatment. These include ingrown toenails, moles and warts, athlete's foot, ringworm and other fungal growths, corns and calluses.

Insect Bites: The pain and itching due to insect bites can be relieved by daily applications of Aloe Vera. This may be due to the deep, penetrating qualities of the gel.

Poison Oak, Poison Ivy: This annoying dermatological plague has been the bane of campers and other outdoor people for years. While time is the best natural way to heal, at least Aloe Vera can work effectively to reduce the itching.

Arthritis: This disabling disease, unfortunately, is one illness still in search of a cure. While Aloe Vera will not cure the problem, many believe that drinking the Aloe Vera juice helps to relieve the pain.

Cuts and Minor Abrasions: There are numerous Aloe Vera uses, should you cut yourself. The gel, with its anti-bacterial qualities, is especially important in the event of a cut. In addition, the Aloe Vera's calcium helps to promote the healing process by fostering blood clotting.

Nose Congestion: Many people use Aloe Vera as a decongestant. Patients treated with Aloe Vera were able to breathe and smell with greater ease.

Bed Wetting: The Soviets, who have conducted most of the extensive research about Aloe Vera, claim to have reduced the incidence of bed wetting after daily injections of aloe extract were given to a number of children. According to one report, the bed wetting completely disappeared after seven to ten injections. We must, in good faith, point out, however, that we do not know of any

American tests in this area. Do not administer Aloe Vera in this fashion to a child without guidance by a physician.

Joint and Muscle Aches: Because of Aloe Vera's deep penetrating powers, it works wonders on severe joint and muscle pains.

Hearing Dysfunctions: Again, researchers in the Soviet Union are credited with the use of Aloe Vera in auditory dysfunction. In their research, the scientists found that Aloe Vera prevented the deterioration of remaining nerve fibers in cases where a patient was suffering from hearing loss.

Tuberculosis: Both South American and Soviet scientists have discovered that the plant's extract seems to stop or slow the growth of the tuberculin bacteria. The Russians reported that results for those patients who had been inhalents of Aloe Vera extract were impressive. They coughed less and the other signs of this terrible disease ceased.

Anemia: The iron contained in the gel can be used effectively against anemia. When added to iron preparations, the gel reduced the irritating effect of the iron on the gastrointestinal system.

There are literally hundreds of other ailments that Aloe Vera, in one form or another, is alleged to have helped cure. Beware, not all of this has been documented and there have, indeed, been cases of exaggeration by people who have not really understood the importance of scientific testing. As a result, there is some, if not a lot, of validity to many of the claims by critics who detract from the legitimate research now taking place. Aloe Vera, while still a plant of mystery, is touted by many as the cure-all. It isn't. That's why it is so important to seek medical attention for any of the ailments Aloe Vera is supposed to help cure. It is possible your physician will recommend some sort of Aloe Vera treatment, but never take it on yourself to diagnose a problem.

aloe vera:

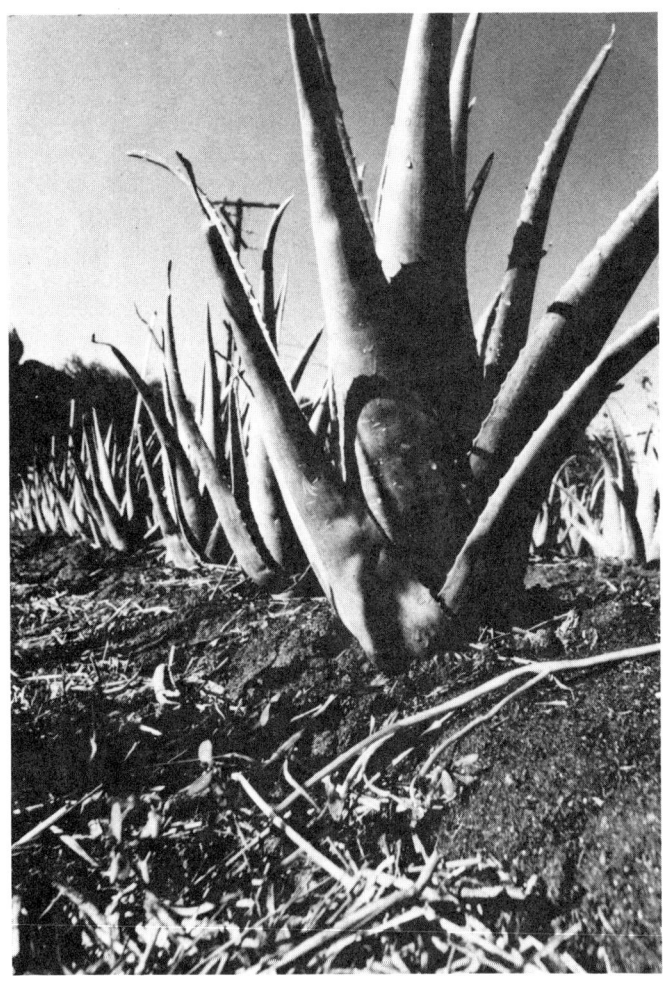

―――――――――――――――the miracle plant

athletic injuries

Aloe Vera as a treatment and as a preventative of athletic injury has recently received increased attention. The best testimonial we have found in favor of Aloe Vera as a method of treatment is by Chuck Piper, Ph.D., former head football and baseball coach for Victor Valley College in Victorbill, California. We've taken the liberty of reprinting it here:

When Aloe Vera products were recommended for my personal health problems, I was very skeptical. My first reaction was, "You've got to be kidding." It just sounded too good to be true.

Thank goodness, common sense prevailed. I started to use the products, and as I heard more and more individuals expound on the benefits they were receiving from using Aloe Vera, plus the benefits I was experiencing, I had to admit Aloe Vera did the job.

As I continued to experience better health as a result of using Aloe Vera, the following question kept popping up in my thoughts. If Aloe Vera was doing such a fantastic job for so many people, why wouldn't it work in the prevention and care of athletic injuries? Many of the problems people were combatting in day-to-day living with the use of Aloe Vera were some of the same problems I had faced in caring for the physical well-being of high school and junior college athletes during my twenty-eight years of coaching.

Yet, I was still reluctant to jump on the Aloe Vera bandwagon for athletics until I personally used it in our athletic program and had conducted some additional research.

My research started in our area of Southern California. I fully expected to find a wealth of material, and coaches who were using Aloe Vera for all types of athletic injury problems. Unfortunately, this was not so. As I pored over volumes of readers guide, subject guides, etc., I could find no mention of Aloe Vera's use in athletics. Several coaches had seen and heard of the Aloe Vera plant but knew nothing about Aloe Vera products and their use in injury treatment.

As I expanded my contacts with high school and college coaches in the Midwest, East, Southeast, and several Western states during my summer vacation and a sabbatical leave, I once again found very limited knowledge about Aloe Vera and athletics.

Like the prospector, Mr. Darby, who stopped digging just three feet from one of the largest gold strikes in our country's history, I was ready to call it quits. Then I talked to a coaching friend in Texas who said, "Oh yes, I know about Aloe Vera. I'm sold on it. I have our trainer use it on our football squad. It's worked great for us. It has cut down on our injuries and when a player is injured, such as a sprain, strain, tear, etc., it gets him back to action sooner." Eureka!

Several weeks later, another breakthrough. I found there was an outstanding book, recently published, called, *The Silent Healer, A Modern Study of Aloe Vera,* and it devoted an entire chapter to Aloe Vera and athletics.

I ordered a copy immediately. Being impatient to get the book, I called the author, Bill Coats, R. Ph., several times to discuss Aloe Vera and athletics. I found that Aloe

the miracle plant

Vera was being used by a number of professional football teams, several professional baseball clubs, many Southwestern universities, colleges, and high school athletic programs. It had even been used in the 1976 Olympics at Montreal.

When I received my copy of Coats' book, I found the material to be exceptionally well-documented, with statements from outstanding individuals associated with professional, college, and high school athletics, expressing their complete satisfaction with the use of Aloe Vera in the treatment of athletic injuries.

Yet, something still bothered me. If the above individuals were sold on Aloe Vera, what was the reason or reasons coaches I had talked to throughout the nation did not have more information of Aloe Vera's use in athletics?

I realized why as I reread Chapter 8 in Coats' book, rechecked the areas I had been in and coaches I had talked with.

The reasons appeared to be:

1) Schools using Aloe Vera in athletic care normally employed a qualified athletic trainer on their staff.

Apparently the majority of coaches I had talked with were not so fortunate as to have a qualified athletic trainer on their staff. The standard operating procedure in secondary school athletic programs, in regard to athletic training, is for the assistant coaches to assume the responsibility of athletic trainers. It saves money. In this dual role, the coach is not in every-day contact with other athletic trainers, nor does he usually attend athletic training clinics where he would come in contact with trainers who were using Aloe Vera.

2) Use of Aloe Vera for secondary school athletics was basically restricted to the Southwest.

The Aloe Vera plant from which Aloe Vera products are made is grown on plantations in the fertile soil of the Rio

aloe vera:

Grande Valley of south Texas. You just don't find Aloe Vera plantations in Indiana, New York, or Pennsylvania. I had assumed if a coach was using such a fine product as Aloe Vera for athletic injuries and getting good results, he would share his findings with other coaches, just like he shares ideas on offensive-defensive techniques, fast break patterns, hitting tips, etc. I was wrong.

3) Aloe Vera products are normally marketed by individuals who are engaged in a multi-level marketing business structure.

The coach or coach-trainer relies a great deal on the sporting goods salesman or athletic training supply representative for the latest in new training ideas and products. Multi-level marketing personnel normally do not call on schools in marketing their products.

While the use of Aloe Vera in athletic training has been a well-kept secret, it should not be pushed aside as a Johnny-come-lately or treated as the new kid on the block. The Aloe Vera plant and its tremendous healing properties have been around, known and used by various cultures and societies for more than two thousand three hundred years. It has been through the dedication and efforts of Bill Coats that a stabilization process was perfected, which provides us with products having almost identical properties as the original plant leaves prior to harvesting.

REPORTED USES OF ALOE VERA IN PREVENTION AND TREATMENT OF ATHLETIC INJURIES

Ankle Sprains — Elbow Bruises — Astro Toe

This is an area of treatment in athletics that was frustrating to me as a coach. It seemed that once an athlete sprained an ankle, he seemed to be plagued with an ankle problem the rest of the season. No matter how much time he spent in the whirlpool, used ultra-sound, or how good you strapped it, he was always favoring it. In addition, recurrence of swelling and pain was common, and complete recovery only took place after the season, when the ankle could be rested with no stress involved. Therefore, I was very interested in how Aloe Vera could be used in treatment of this type of injury. In my research, I found several different approaches and techniques being used, with each producing excellent results.

When I talked to Don Cochren, head trainer for the Dallas Cowboys, at the Cowboys' pre-season camp recently, he stated he had used Aloe Vera gel to reduce ankle-sprain swelling and pain by wrapping the ankle with a gauze wrap that had been soaked with Aloe Vera gel, then applying an elastic-type bandage loosely and applying ice. Cochren said he had been introduced to Aloe Vera in a rather unique situation. One of their fullbacks had sprained his ankle in an off-season, evening basketball game and had been given some Aloe Vera gel by a friend, who told him that it would reduce the pain. The player took the advice, applied the gel and ice overnight and walked into the training room the next day with no swelling or pain and recommended its use to the Cowboys. Cochren also said he uses Aloe Vera gel in combatting swelling, elbow bruise pain and Astro toe.

Coats reports that Spanky Stephens, University of Texas trainer, uses Aloe Vera gel as starter treatment for all sprains and strains. Stephens freezes the gel and uses it as an ice massage. He then uses a methyl salicylate product, after which he places a cold hydrocollator on the injury with both products under it. This treatment stops the peripheral bleeding and pain. Stephens also makes daily use of Aloe Vera gel in both his hot and cold whirlpools for injured athletes.

Tendinitis

Arm soreness of some type is a common problem with young pitchers during the early part of the baseball season

aloe vera:

and, without proper care, the problem can be compounded and plague the hurler for an entire season. This is especially true in areas where early preseason weather in the months of January and February is cold and nasty. Normally, the young pitcher fails to protect his arm adequately from the elements or fails to warm up properly before hard pitching. The result is usually some form of arm pain due to tendinitis. This happened to one of our community college pitchers this past season during the early part of January.

When he visited a well-known arm specialist, the recommendation was to hang up the glove for the year and let the arm have a complete rest. The pitcher was unwilling to take this advice. While he refrained from throwing hard and doing the regular pitcher's throwing workout, he did keep in shape by running, easy tossing, and, finally, the arm started to respond, yet there was always this touch of painful tendinitis lurking on the surface. One day when talking about his arm tenderness, he asked about using some type of superficial heat to help combat the problem. I then told him some of the stories I had heard concerning the use of Aloe Vera heat lotion for deep pain and muscle soreness. He started to apply the heat lotion several times a day, for a period of approximately two weeks, and reported no arm tenderness whatsoever when he went back to the regular pitcher's workout. In short, his arm responded to the point where he started to take his regular turn in the pitching rotation.

Athlete's Foot

The player should dry his feet thoroughly, then massage Aloe Vera gel into the feet. Make sure the gel is massaged in between the toes and over the callused heel and big toe. Applying the gel over the callus causes the dead skin to slough off naturally, which helps combat the age-old problem of blisters developing under calluses during the season. You may also find that Aloe Vera gel keeps the

the miracle plant

feet soft, which helps if a player has a history of corns. The number of recommended applications of Aloe Vera gel varies from one person to the next. Our former trainer, Willie Pringle, cured a rather difficult case of athlete's foot in three days by applying the gel four to six times per day. After the itching and peeling had subsided, he applied the gel in the morning and evening.

Blisters

In treating blisters, Aloe Vera gel can be used. If the skin is broken, trim as much of the loose skin away as possible and apply the gel generously to the exposed blister area. If possible, leave the area free of bandages and let the player wear a pair of flip-flops so that additional gel can be applied four or five times a day. If there is any danger of dirt getting into the open blister, use a gauze-type protection. When the blister is not broken, and fluid remains under the skin, cut a small opening in the blister, let the fluid drain, squirt as much of the gel as possible into the opening, and cover the area with a gauze pad saturated with gel. As soon as the healing process begins, and the tenderness under the blister subsides, trim off as much of the loose skin as possible and continue treatment as I previously mentioned.

Sunburn

For coaches who have players reporting with deep sunburns, Aloe Vera gel or Aloe Vera lotion may be the answer. The problem of sunburn really hit home with me when I coached our community college women's softball squad. Since we are within one hundred miles of some of Southern California's best beach and resort areas, I was continually faced with the problem of a player having to miss a practice because of sunburn.

One Monday during the middle of our season, my only catcher (a blonde with light complexion) showed up after a weekend in Palm Springs, red as a beet and burnt to a crisp. I wanted to be sympathetic and let her skip practice,

aloe vera:

but we had a game the next day and I needed her at practice. When I told her to loosen up and get her catching gear on, she complained about the intense sunburn pain. I remembered I had a bottle of Aloe Vera gel in the glove compartment of my truck; I had heard how it helped burns. I got the gel, rubbed it on her face, arms and legs, then had a couple of the girls put gel on her back, shoulders and stomach. Darn if she didn't come back and say, "Coach, the heat and burning sensation is gone." She put the gear on and worked out with no ill effects.

Since coaching that squad, Aloe Vera suntan lotion has been marketed; it blocks harmful sun rays yet allows the individual to get a good tan.

Additional Aloe Vera Uses

Bill Hicks, head football coach at Paris High School in Paris, Texas, says that in addition to making use of Aloe Vera gel for sprains, elbow bruises, hamstring pulls, and thigh bruises, his trainer uses the gel with whirlpool treatments, massage and ultra-sound. Additionally, Hicks' team members use Aloe Vera gel for the treatment of cuts and burns received from playing on both natural grass and artificial turf. I was especially interested in his approach to the use of Aloe Vera gel in the prevention of injuries. Coaches are faced with the age-old problem of muscle tightness among their players prior to kick-off or regulation play. Many times it takes a player anywhere from five to ten minutes to get loose, but if he gets hit hard early in the contest, an injury can result. Hicks has his players (especially his fullbacks) rub Aloe Vera gel on their legs one-half hour prior to game time. He has found that it helps loosen their leg muscles and has cut down on injuries early in the game.

The benefits described here are not the only benefits a coach or trainer will achieve from the use of Aloe Vera. I believe we have only scratched the surface in regard to aloe's use in athletics. Give it a try.

―――――――――――――――― *the miracle plant*

25 questions

1. Exactly what is Aloe Vera?

Aloe Vera is a leaf succulent that boasts more than two hundred species of the plant. About one hundred fifty of them are in the family *Lilaceae*, which happens to be the same botanical classification as lilies, some types of tulips, onions, asparagus and more. It's grown in various places around the world, mostly in dry and hot areas. In the United States, it is cultivated predominantly in southern Texas.

2. Why all of the media attention all of a sudden about a plant?

There's nothing sudden about it. Man learned to appreciate the miracles of the Aloe Vera plant before recorded history. Some of the earliest references to it appear in the *Bible*.

3. What stimulates current interest in the plant?

That's hard to say, but probably the interest in natural products for both health and cosmetic purposes. The consuming public is becoming more aware of the plant's benefits and, as a result, more companies are being formed to meet those demands.

4. Is Aloe Vera a medicine?

The Food and Drug Administration does not recognize Aloe Vera as a medicine. Whatever it's called, though, the

aloe vera:

plant has various curative powers described earlier in this booklet. As more and more research takes place, there is little doubt that the FDA will also recognize some — if not all — of the plant's benefits.

5. *What part of the Aloe Vera plant is used?*

Many parts are used although, by far, the most popular is the gel itself, which comes from inside the spiny leaves.

6. *In what part of the world is knowledge about the Aloe Vera plant supposed to have originated?*

As with many of man's discoveries, it was first noticed as a plant of wonder in the southern part of the cradle of civilization, Egypt. References to it can be found on pyramid walls.

7. *Was this civilization the first to recognize the medicinal value of the Aloe Vera plant?*

No. As far as we can determine, its first pharmaceutical use came in Sumeria about 1750 B.C.

8. *Will Aloe Vera increase sexual potency?*

No. But it does have many important vitamins and minerals that can help you develop a healthy life. A healthy body can benefit many facets of day-to-day living, including sexually fulfilling relationships.

9. *Is Aloe Vera always the answer?*

No. As with any treatment, you should not begin any program without first consulting your family physician or other health professional.

10. *For what injury does Aloe Vera seem to have the most value?*

That's difficult to say. There are many people who have reported that Aloe Vera products have helped everything from hemorrhoids to arthritis. Most of the publicized research, however, has been in the field of burn treatment.

11. *If Aloe Vera is so good, why doesn't the Food and Drug Administration (FDA) recognize its many medical benefits?*

That's a good question. The time may come when the FDA will recognize that there is a place for Aloe Vera products in the medical marketplace. As with all drugs, the procedure for verification is long and difficult. Note that this isn't necessarily bad. It just means that the time has not yet come when applications are viewed favorably.

12. *What is being done by Aloe Vera companies to promote the benefits of this plant?*

Many companies have formed the National Aloe Science Council, which not only promotes Aloe Vera but also helps to regulate the marketplace. This is not to say that those companies that don't belong to this umbrella organization are not striving to the same end. It just means that some companies have taken it upon themselves to join together for what they see as the common good.

13. *That's all fine and dandy. But how does Aloe Vera help me as a person who suffers extreme problems with bursitis?*

That's hard to say without knowing your medical history. But it is possible to point to numerous statements by lay people as well as medical professionals — all of whom contend that rubbing the gel of the Aloe Vera plant over the affected area will help to relieve the pain.

14. *How does rubbing it over a sore spot do anything?*

Aloe Vera has unique penetrating powers, which makes it a useful transportation vehicle, if you will. There are athletic trainers, for example, who crush aspirin over an injury — say an ankle sprain — and then rub Aloe Vera over the aspirin. One well-known coach says the Aloe Vera helps the aspirin to penetrate the skin at the point of the injury.

15. *What about arthritis? This treatment sounds like it may help me.*

Again, because your medical condition may be unique, it's not possible to promise any miracle results. Certainly, in consultation with your physician, though, it may be worth a try.

16. *I've had ulcers for years. A friend of mine who works in the fields in south Texas has been drinking the juice for years. He claims it has helped his stomach and controls his ulcer.*

This is not a unique treatment. It's something worth asking your physician about. Keep in mind, though, that some people do have a severe reaction from ingesting the juice. It's rare, but there are those who may become sick to their stomach or contract diarrhea. Obviously, if these conditions persist, you should discontinue drinking the juice and consult your doctor for an appropriate alternate treatment.

17. *Is it true that Aloe Vera cosmetics are better than other types?*

Aloe Vera companies obviously think so and there are numerous consumers who would say that. In fact, Aloe Vera products are becoming so popular among cosmetic companies that some of the major cosmetic manufacturers are including some Aloe Vera in many of their products. Keep in mind, though, that it is extremely important to know the percentage of Aloe Vera in a given product. If there is less than 70 percent Aloe Vera in a cosmetic item, you should reconsider its purchase.

18. *What if I were to go out and buy an Aloe Vera plant and take its gel out for use in my cosmetics? Would this be the same as purchasing Aloe Vera products?*

First, you probably won't know the chemistry of the cosmetics you have. This could lead to a severe skin reaction. Second, even if you did understand the chemistry, there is one important factor to consider. Aloe Vera gel must be stabilized to be preserved. This stabilization process is a closely guarded trade secret at many companies. Without stabilization, Aloe Vera can go bad and cause many side effects.

19. *Can I lose weight with Aloe Vera?*

In a way, you can. If you begin a diet program, Aloe Vera juice and some of the other food products that are derived from the Aloe Vera plant will offer most of a normal, healthy adult's required vitamins and minerals. This is extremely important in a diet program.

20. *Where can I purchase Aloe Vera food products, including the juice?*

In most health food stores around the country. Aloe Vera products are becoming more popular as more is written about them.

21. *I live in California and enjoy my days at the beach. How can Aloe Vera products be of use to me?*

One of the most effective Aloe Vera items on the market is sunscreen or suntan oil containing Aloe Vera. If already sunburned, you can apply Aloe Vera cream to your body for relief. It provides an enormous amount of relief.

22. *In my town in upstate Illinois, there is a lot of poison ivy to which I am allergic. Can Aloe Vera help me?*

It really can't do anything for your allergies, but it does have value for relieving the itch. By applying the cream

aloe vera:

regularly, you can relieve the discomfort of poison ivy. The same goes for related plant afflictions, like poison oak.

23. *Is there a complete list available of medical conditions that Aloe Vera is supposed to help cure?*

Yes. The list was compiled by Carol Miller Kent in her research work on Aloe Vera, published in 1979 in Arlington, Virginia. For those who do not have access to this fine research paper, the list is reprinted here: ". . . a whole spectrum of skin disorders including thermal, chemical and friction burns, scald; sunburn; radium, X-ray and other radiation burns, ulcers and blisters; diaper and heat rashes, prickly heat, razor burn, windburn, turf burns and abrasions; wasp, bee and fly stings; mosquito and other insect bites; poison ivy and poison oak; allergic reactions; eruptions and rashes of childhood diseases; chafed, chapped or scaly skin, and chapped lips; dandruff, eczema, dermatitis, impetigo, seborrhea, psoriasis, and uriticaria; body and bed sores; body odor; skin cancer; herpes zoster (shingles); sore or cracked nipples in nursing mothers; ingrown toenails; pimples, acne, blemishes, brown or white "liver spots" (chloasma), sensitive moles, pedunculated fibromas, and warts; cuts, contusions, lacerations, wet or dry lesions; chronic ulcers; boils and abscesses; canker sores, cold sores, fever blisters, herpes simplex (both oral and lip), minor sore throat, mouth irritations, denture sores, gingivitis, tonsillitis, mouth and gum diseases, staphyloccocal infections; conjunctivitis, styles, corneal ulcers, and cataracts; puncture wounds and infected pierced ears; athlete's foot, ringworm and other fungi, pruritus ani, valvae, balnea, essential pruritis, vaginal yeast infections; venereal sores, muscle cramps, strains, sprains, bruises, swelling, soreness, tendinitis and bursitis; loss of hair (alopecia).

the miracle plant

Taken internally, Aloe Vera is said to alleviate headache, insomnia, bad breath; stomach disorders, indigestion, heartburn, hyper-acidity gastritis, peptic and duodenal ulcers; colitis, hemorrhoids, kidney and urinary tract infections; prostatitis, fistulas and inflamed cysts; diabetes; high blood pressure, rheumatism and arthritis. It is claimed to eliminate pinworms and other parasites, correct functional infertility caused by amenorrhea, and reverse any imbalance caused or amplified by excess acid or sugar ingestion."

24. *If it's so good, why doesn't my family doctor recommend it?*

Many doctors are recommending it. In one of the testimonial letters printed in the next section of this booklet, you can find a letter by a dermatologist who is extremely interested in finding out more about Aloe Vera's unique properties. Keep in mind, as well, that the list quoted above refers to known uses of Aloe Vera throughout history. It does not mean that all of them can be substantiated in modern times.

25. *If Aloe Vera is so good for humans, it must be good for pets, as well.*

That's true. The gel can be used in treatment of an open wound or burn, for example. In addition, Aloe Vera can be used as a de-fleaing agent.

aloe vera:

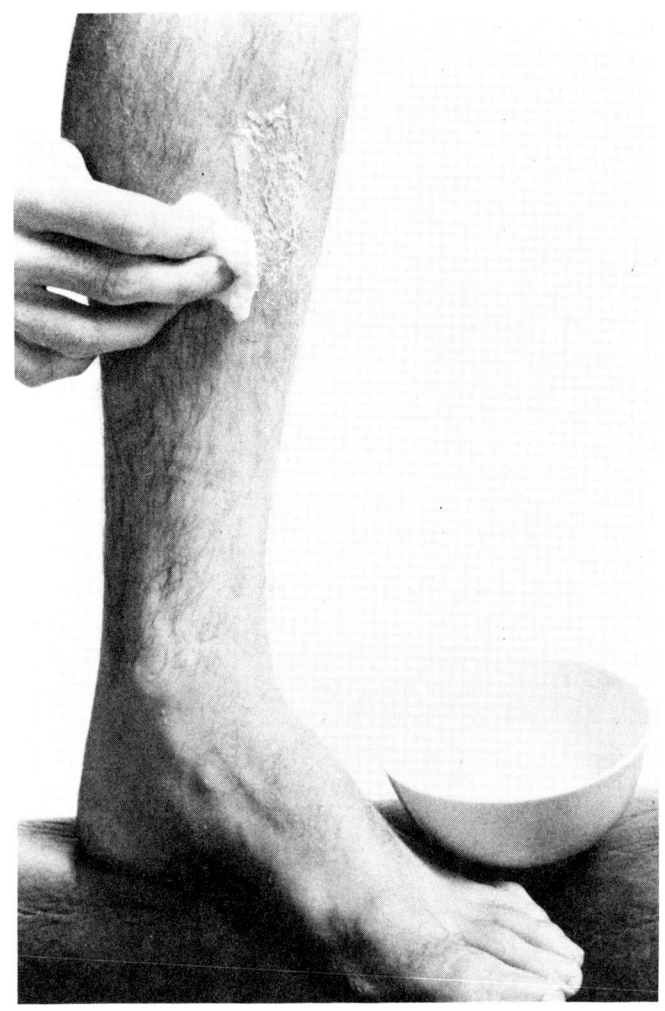

_____the miracle plant

three case histories

Pat Proskin of Antioch, Illinois, was working in her kitchen when she accidentally burned her lower arm on a hot oven. She had no remedy in her home, except for the succulent growing in a pot in her living room. A friend had given her a cutting from her succulent and since this type of plant does not require a lot of special care, it did not take long until Mrs. Proskin owned a medium-sized Aloe Vera plant. (By the way, Antioch is north of Chicago on the Wisconsin border. Midwesterners know how cold this area can get in the winter, which in itself is a testament to the vitality of the Aloe Vera plant.) This is Mrs. Proskin's story:

"After I burned myself, I took a cutting from my Aloe Vera plant and squeezed some of the gel out of the leaf. I don't know how I knew that this might help me. Maybe a friend told me about Aloe Vera's unique healing powers. Anyway, I rubbed the gel on the affected area. My only immediate benefit was a bit of relief from the excruciating pain. Of course, that probably would have been the benefit from any liquid substance.

"But I decided to see how beneficial the gel would be. A friend of mine has a plant at work and so, every hour during the working day for the next two and a half days, I would rub the gel on the burn. When I returned home in the evening, I would continue this sort of treatment.

aloe vera:

"After two and a half days, the burn, which was rather severe, was not bothering me anymore. In fact, the scar from the burn was minimal, hardly noticeable. I have never seen results so quickly as I did after applying the Aloe Vera gel. Since then, I have told all my friends about Aloe Vera and I continue to use it when I cut or burn myself. Nobody can tell me it doesn't work. I saw with my own eyes, on my own body, that it offers fast results."

Mrs. Proskin recently broke her arm and will be rubbing the gel on her arm when her cast comes off (at this writing, it still is on her arm). She says she is confident that the gel will relieve any pain she might have.

"I would have been dead without Aloe Vera. No question about it," says J.M. Hayner of Shreveport, Louisiana. In 1976, Hayner, a retired geologist, developed a severe case of bilateral scleroderma, a disease that stiffens skin tissue, often causing the skin to develop ulcers. Hayner's lower legs were so ulcerated that he considered taking his life rather than endure further pain. Certainly, no relief from his excruciatingly painful situation was in sight. Hayner's dermatologist, Dr. Albert Irving Clark, also of Shreveport, had tried every known cure, including wet casts, honey, biozyme, grandulex, gold leaf, and other treatments. But Hayner's condition continued to worsen. It was at this point that Hayner discovered his own cure: Aloe Vera. Learning of Aloe Vera's miracle wonders through friends, Hayner asked Clark about the substance. Clark was unfamiliar with Aloe Vera but made inquiries. "Frankly, at the time, I felt his situation was hopeless. I would have tried anything," says Clark.

Hayner was hospitalized and an Aloe Vera poultice applied to his ulcers for eight hours a day. Hayner also drank Aloe Vera in liquid form. The results were astonishing, both Hayner and Clark agree. Within months after the treatment, the ulcers began to heal. And Hayner, who had been unable to walk because of the ulcers, began to

the miracle plant

walk again. With the continuing application of Aloe Vera, Hayner's ulcers all but disappeared a year later.

Clark was so astonished at his patient's progress that he wrote the following to the maker of the Aloe Vera product used in the treatment:

I have been very impressed with the value of Aloe Vera in this case, when I consider the numerous modalities used prior to Aloe Vera without any results; when I consider that other dermatologists to whom I sent him did nothing; when I consider that everyone I have spoken to offered me no hope. I can say that the use of Aloe Vera has cured this man of the severe ulcerations that went with the bilateral scleroderma. When I consider the man also has diabetes, hypertension, elevated cholesterol, and rheumatoid arthritis as concomitant diseases, I can wholeheartedly state without equivocation that the only thing that healed extensive ulcerations of both lower extremities was the use of Aloe Vera . . .

Today, Hayner is a hale and hearty man who recently celebrated his seventy-fourth birthday. Although his condition is cured, he still uses Aloe Vera lotion on his legs every other day "to keep the skin soft," he says.

This testimonial is based on information drawn from *The Silent Healer* by Bill Coats and on interviews with J.M. Hayner and Dr. Albert Irving Clark.

"Maybe there's something in this," Patsy England of Dallas said to herself ten years ago. England was referring to Aloe Vera. After a lifetime of suffering skin so dry that it made her look twice her age, England, at forty-two, was ready to try something different. For twenty years, she says her life had been "a constant battle with body skin, bumps, flaking, irritations." Doctors had told her that her body was unable to produce normal amounts of natural moisture. Their only solution: move to a very humid climate.

aloe vera:

England adds, "After years of using top brand, expensive products and following experts' advice, gained as advertising director of several prestigious department stores, I did not believe the promise of any cosmetic product."

England's discovery of Aloe Vera came about through observing the results her father obtained for his arthritis by drinking the gel. At that point in her life, England's skin was not only painfully dry, but her forehead was covered with brown liver spots.

Shortly after beginning a skin regimen with Aloe Vera products, England's skin began to look and feel different. "Within the first year, the brown spots began to fade, eventually totally disappearing, and have not returned, even with annual sun exposure," England says. "But most important . . . my facial skin is no longer dry. A fact! Gradually switching to products with less and less oil, I now follow a prescriptive routine that even contains non-oily products . . . all of which has kept my skin soft, moist and younger looking than it was twenty years ago . . . The constant aloe penetration in all of the products on my skin has created miracles. My father and friends constantly recognize this fact, but find it hard to believe it is the same skin."

This testimonial is based on information drawn from The Silent Healer *by Bill Coats and on an interview with Patsy England.*

In the next section, you'll find a wide variety of testimonial letters from people all over the country who have written to Aloe Vera companies. Universally, the reaction is positive toward the wonders of the plant.

Paging through the letters submitted by various companies provides an understanding of how people from all walks of life feel about Aloe Vera.

testimonial letters

Dear Sir:
We have been using the Aloe Vera juice bottled by your company and we like the taste better than that of other companies. We use a great deal of it as my father has cancer of the colon and this gives him more relief than anything he has taken. The doctor has been quite pleased with the way he is doing since taking the juice. We just pray it may heal him.

Mrs. Robert T.
Vandalie, Ohio

Dear Sirs:
I hope you can be of assistance in my research. As part of my residency in dermatology, I will be giving a lecture on non-prescription medications and would like to include your products in my lecture. Patients occasionally ask about aloe products and I have no answers. Please send me information on your products . . . Since some patients swear by aloe products, this will greatly help us.

Earl R., M.D.
Long Beach, California

Dear Sirs:
For 10 years, I have suffered with an allergy that leaves blisters in my nose and they run to my lip. They are very painful and look horrible. I have used everything I could

aloe vera:

find and have spent lots of money on them — but nothing helped.

About two months ago, I started sneezing and here they came. It was bad, bad, bad! I went into a drug store and asked the druggist if he could suggest anything. He started naming everything I had tried. As I was walking out the door, he called to me and gave me a sample of your Aloe Vera product. In two days, the blisters were almost gone!

Bobbye S.
Austin, Texas

Dear Sir:

Would you please sell your Aloe Vera ointment to me on a direct basis? Thought you might like to know it works fantastic for clearing up skin problems on animals as well as problem ears.

Berdeen P.
North Bergen, New Jersey

Dear Sirs:

I have had the pleasure of using your product for a number of years. Since it has no menthol in it, and does have the Aloe Vera gel, I find it is the only lip balm I can use that doesn't dry out my lips, and does promote healing of a split that I get each winter in my lower lip.

Thank you very much.

Father Thomas S.
South Carolina

Dear Sirs:

My wife has suffered for many years with an irritating rash that has developed after exposing her skin to the hot sunshine. She has always taken the sun in moderate doses, and never allowed her skin to become burnt. Whilst taking a holiday in Italy recently, my wife suffered this rash once again and our holiday was in danger of

the miracle plant

spoiling . . . After two applications of your wonderful lotion, all my wife's miseries have disappeared along with the rash.

Yours very sincerely,
John E. B.
London, England

Dear Sir:

I am writing to tell you of my experience with your Aloe Vera drink. I have many canker sores in my mouth which my doctor says will take four to six weeks to heal. I began drinking Aloe Vera drink. I would swish it around my mouth, then drink it. I have been using it ever since. My sores have healed in four days. I could hardly believe it. Also, since taking the drink, my skin has become clearer and younger looking.

Marguerite R.
Indianapolis, Indiana

Gentlemen:

I had to write and tell you how highly I think of your product . . . My hair and skin are very fair and have been since I was a child. In fact, a pediatrician once advised my parents to treat me during summers as though I were albino: long sleeves, long pants, and sunshading hats were to be worn at all times. Thankfully, my sensible parents ignored this counsel; still, I could never remain in the sun for long without risking severe sunburn. I never in my life had anything like a tan until, one summer on Cape Cod, I discovered another of your products . . . which had the ingratiating property of not only healing the sunburn pain overnight, but transforming the burn, after one or two applications, into a moist, non-peeling tan . . .

. . . the gel is the best after-shave preparation I've ever used . . . Now I can shave daily without irritation, razor

aloe vera:

burn or "dry" acne. The gel not only seems to stop the bleeding of nicks and cuts almost immediately, but heals them thoroughly by shaving-time the next morning . . . Several years ago, I had two cysts removed; the lesions never healed properly, and particularly in dry weather, from time to time became inflamed and reopened. Two weeks of application of the gel to the lesions has effectively seen their complete disappearance, with scars much smaller than the surgeon told me to expect.

In the summer, I am plagued with dry and unruly hair — not a terrible problem I admit, so I never gave it much thought. But being a faithful user of the aloe gel for sunburn symptoms, I could not help noticing the effect of aloe on the body hair and my chest and arms, which became soft rather than dry and wiry. I tried aloe gel as a grooming agent for my hair. It's terrific . . . my hair stays in shape while staying soft and conditioned.

Patrick M.
Westport, Connecticut

Dear Sir:

I went to the beach on Monday, got too much sun, and by Friday I could hardly walk. I had tried everything I could find in this small town. Nothing would help, not even the two doctor's prescriptions I had . . . A friend told me of your gel. She said to put it on my legs and take vitamin C daily. I put the gel on my legs, took the vitamin C and was able to sleep for the first night. The next morning my legs were one half the size as the night before, and no pain. I then put on more gel and took more vitamin C, and by that night I was able to wear hose, shoes and attend a wedding. This was my first experience.

On Sunday, my son got a bad scrape on his side — about a two-inch scrape. I put the gel on the wound along, with a bandage; the next morning I did this again.

the miracle plant

That night the skin was back over the scrape. This was unreal, I simply could not believe this could work so fast. This was my second experience.

I never want to be without this gel. This is the greatest stuff I have ever used. It's just great.

Carol H.
Lockhart, Alabama

Dear Sir:

This letter is long overdue and so is the thanks. I just wanted to make sure that your product really did work for me.

This Friday will be exactly one month since I first bought and used this on a very severe itching rash on my forearms. At first it was only a small area. Soon it began to spread over my hands and fingers, and almost up to my elbows.

When I bought your product I started to use it faithfully that same day, every four hours or as soon as the itching was more than I could stand. It relieved the itching, and the relief lasted much longer than all the other (medications).

After the second week, the results were amazing. By the second week the rash was clearing up. By the third week, the itching was gone and the rash began to fade. All this week, I have not used it. The itching has stopped and the rash is just barely visible and still fading.

Elizabeth Z.
Round Lake Park, Illinois

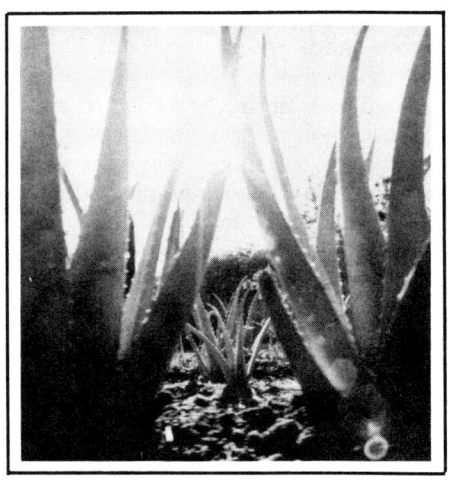